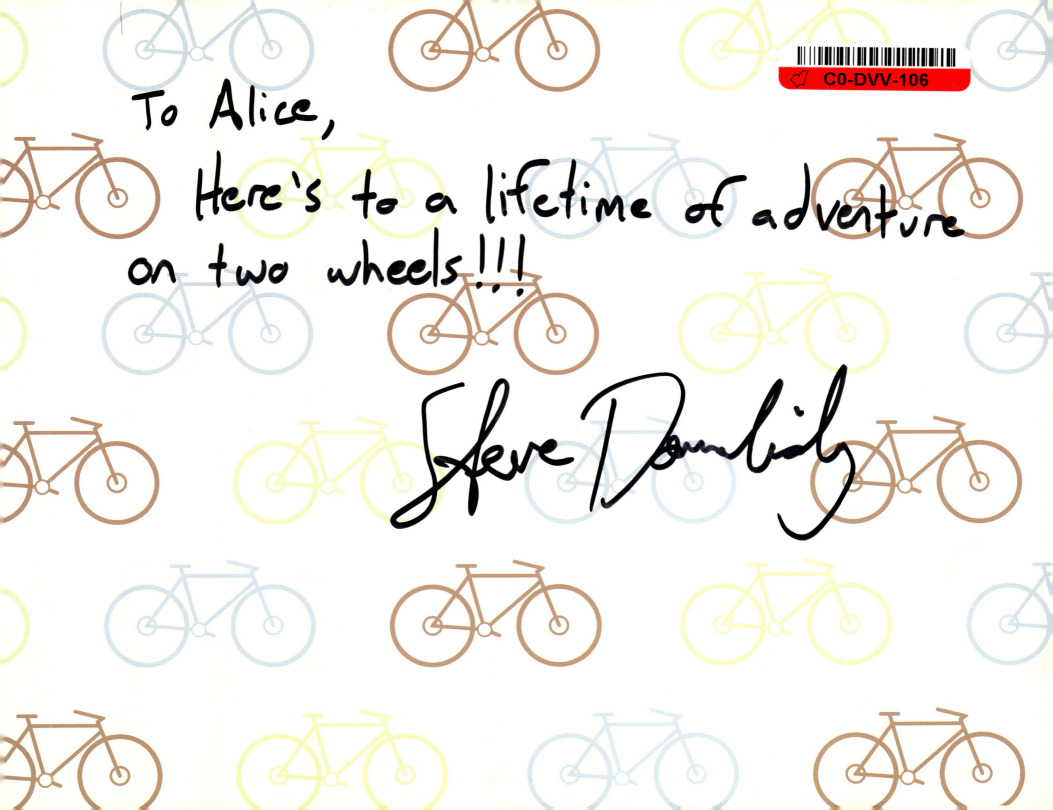

To Alice,
    Here's to a lifetime of adventure
on two wheels!!!

Steve Donnelly

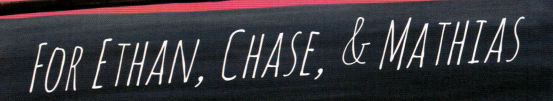

For Ethan, Chase, & Mathias

Library of Congress LCCN Number 2018902572 •
ISBN 978-0-9998996-0-1 (Hardback) [1. Juvenile - Fiction.
2. Cycling - Fiction. 3. Animals - Fiction] • Printed in China
10 9 8 7 6 5 4 3 2 1

A BIKE FOR YOU

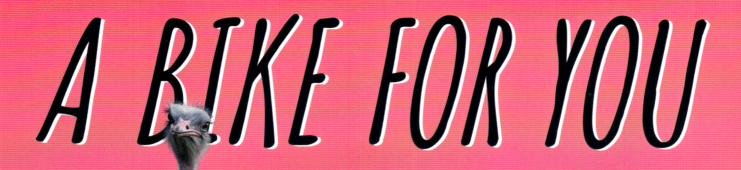

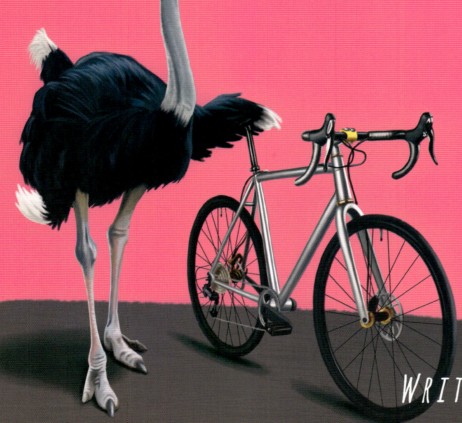

WRITTEN BY STEVE DOMAHIDY

ILLUSTRATED BY ROB SNOW

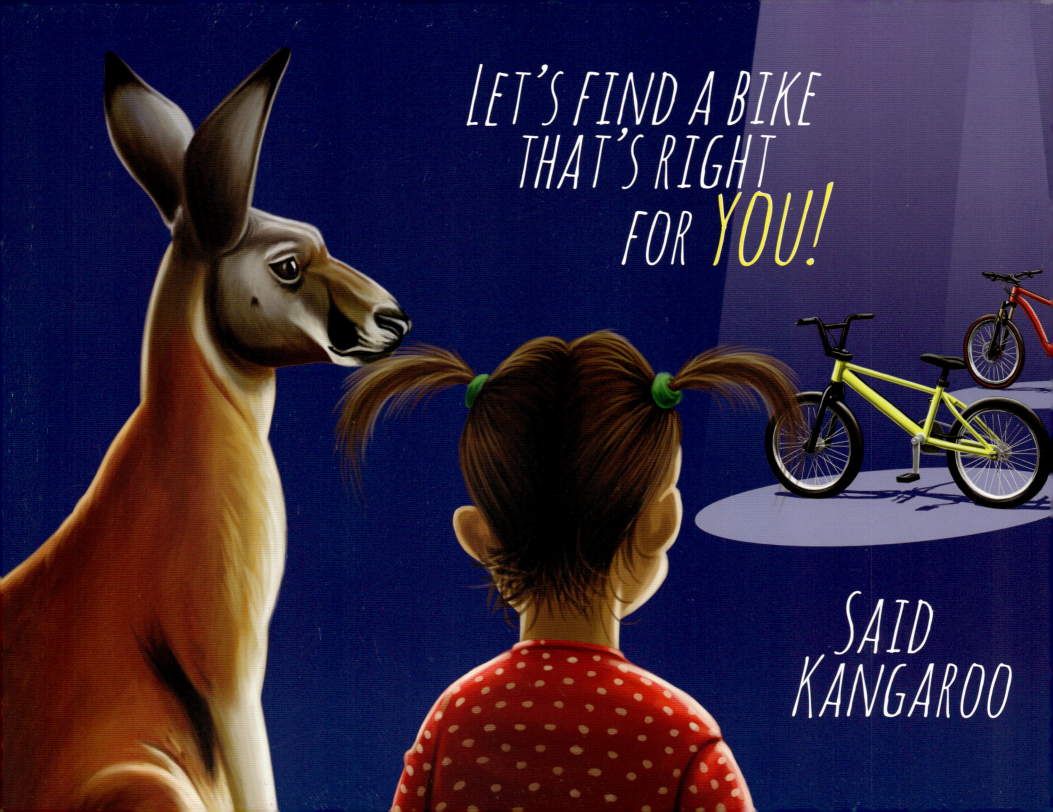

"Let's find a bike that's right for YOU!" said Kangaroo

There are so many different KINDS for different people with different MINDS

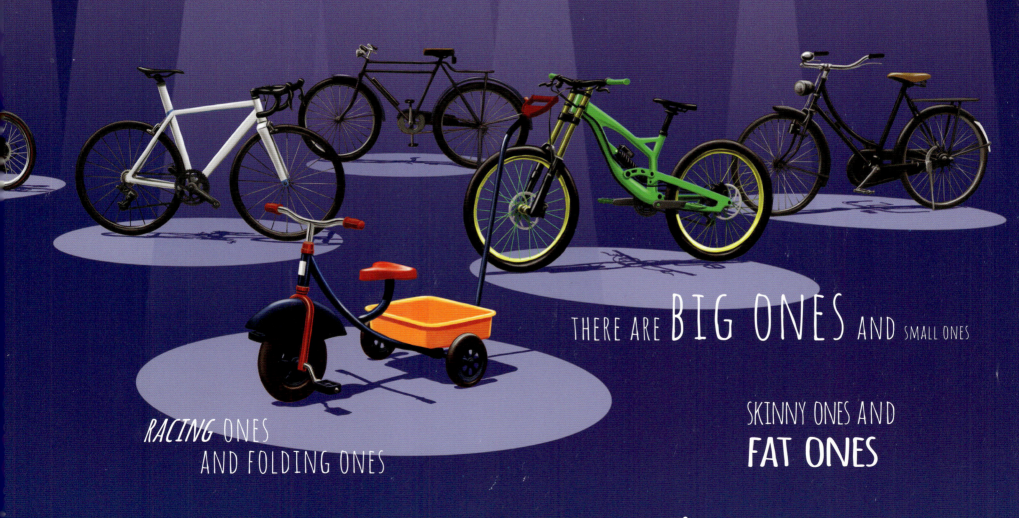

There are BIG ONES and small ones

RACING ONES AND FOLDING ONES

SKINNY ONES AND FAT ONES

AND SO MANY OTHER ONES I CAN'T KEEP TRACK OF

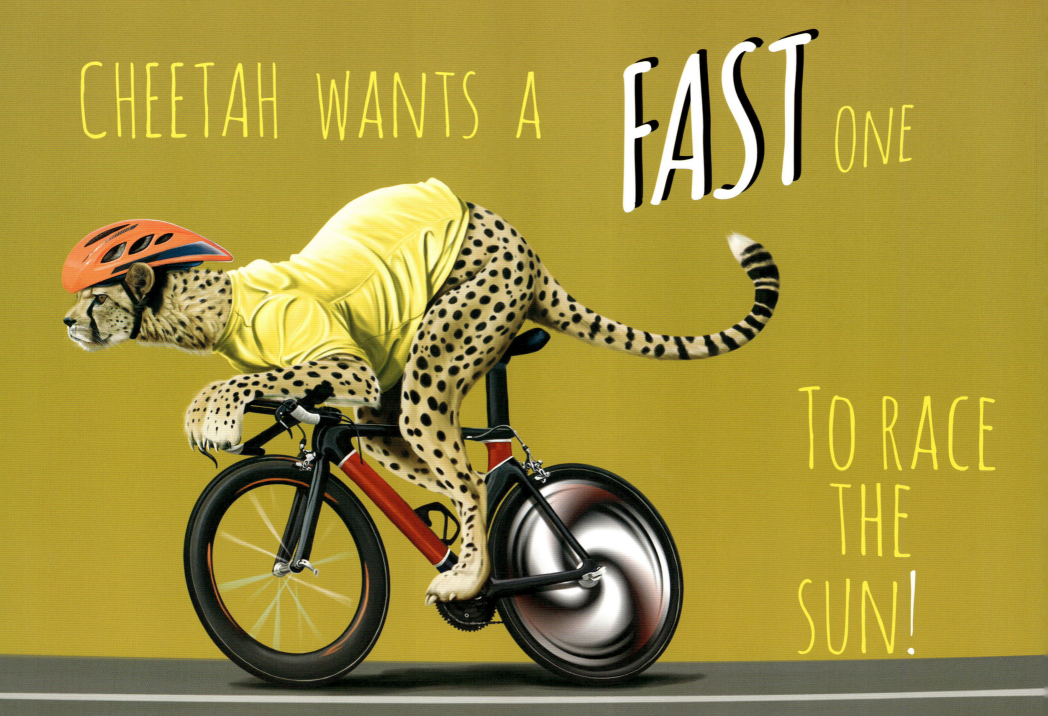

Cheetah wants a **FAST** one

To race the sun!

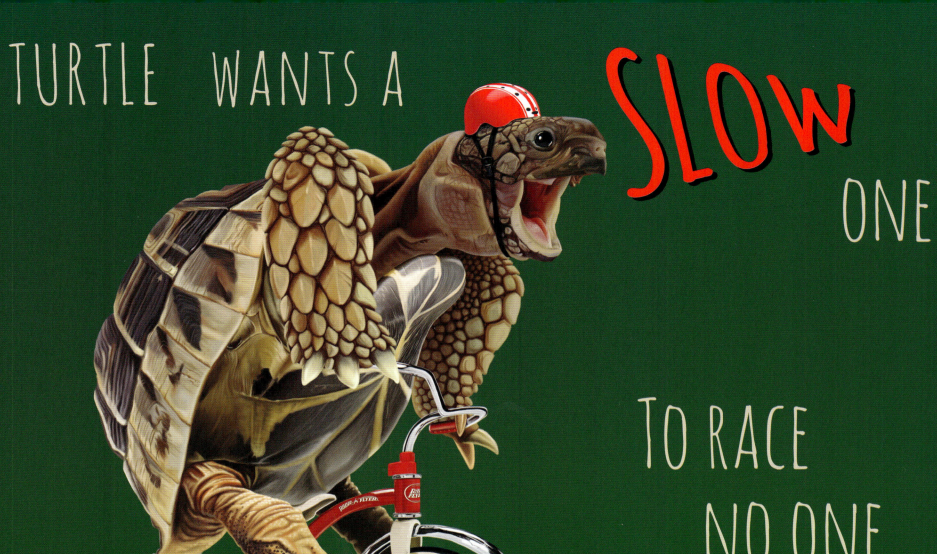

WOLF TAKES HIS ON A TRAIL WITH BUMPS

MONKEY
TAKES
HERS
ON ONE
WITH

JUMPS

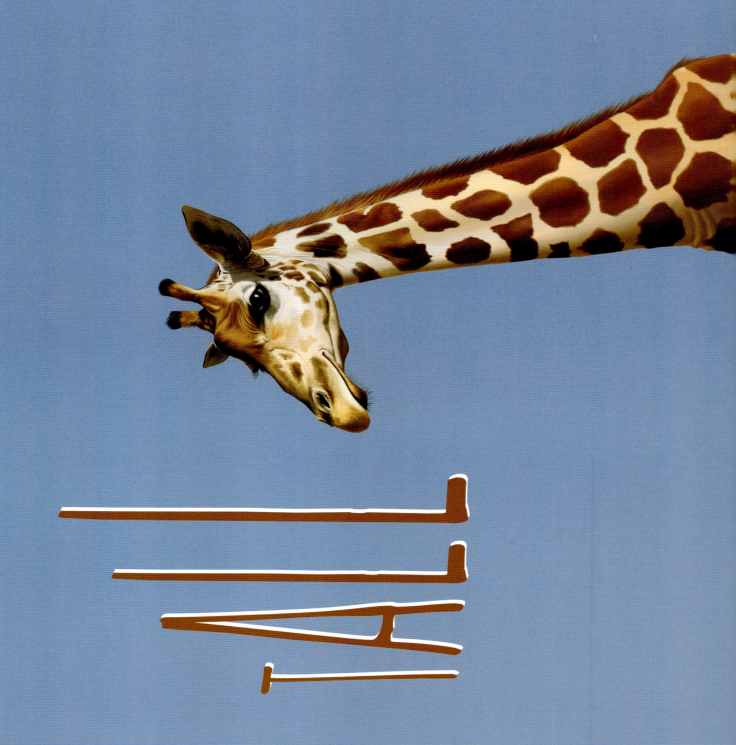

GIRAFFE NEEDS ONE THAT'S

TALL

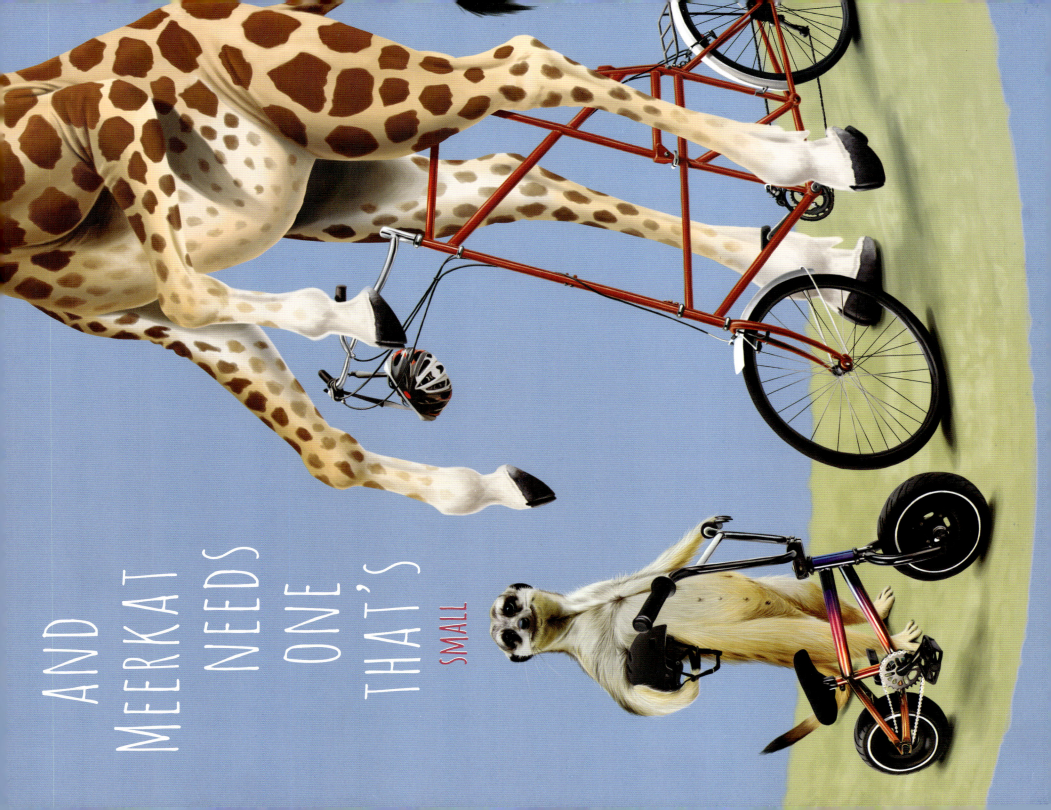

AND MEERKAT NEEDS ONE THAT'S SMALL

RABBIT HAS ONE

THAT NEEDS A

PUSH

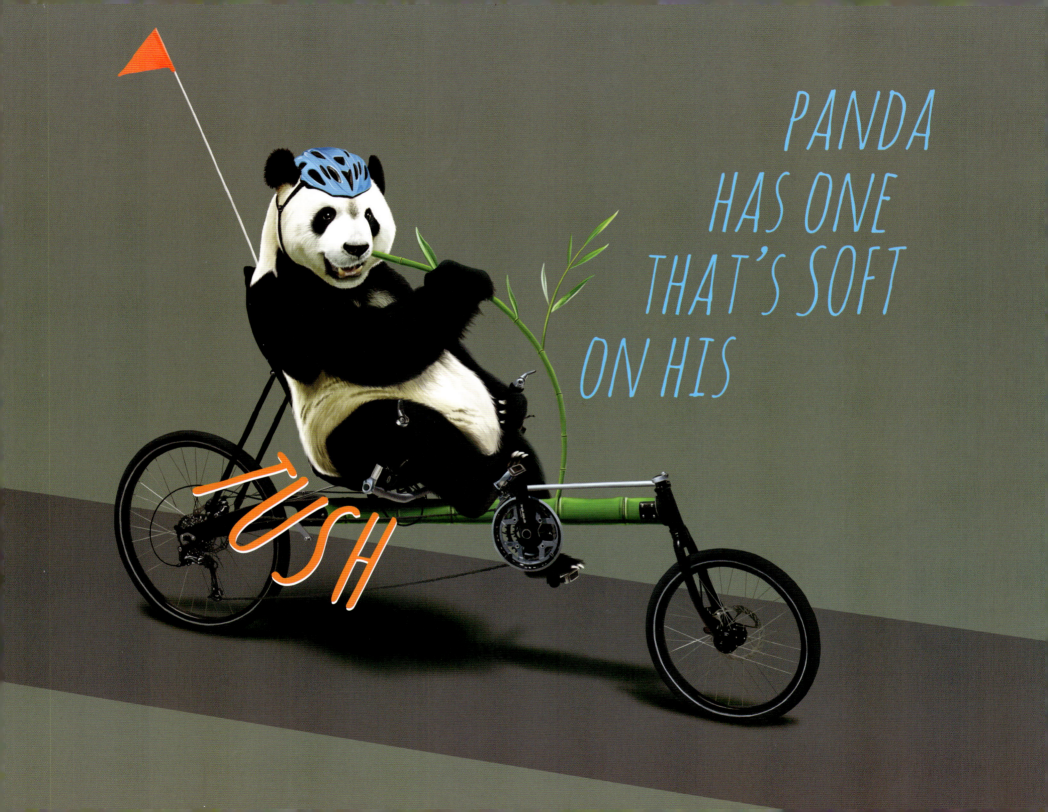

PANDA
HAS ONE
THAT'S SOFT
ON HIS

TUSH

Sometimes you need a bike to get you through

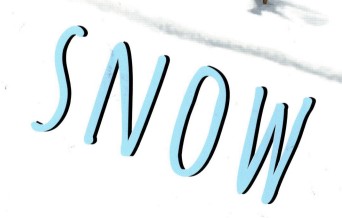

SNOW

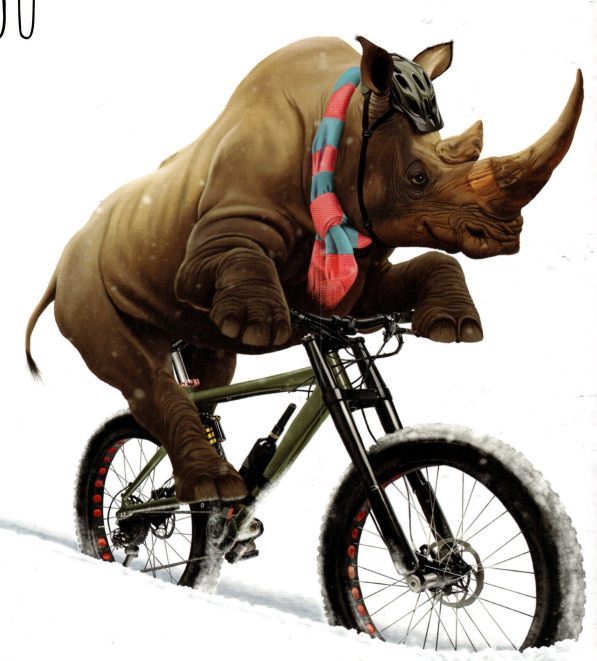

AND SOMETIMES YOU'RE SOMEONE

WHO'S ON THE GO

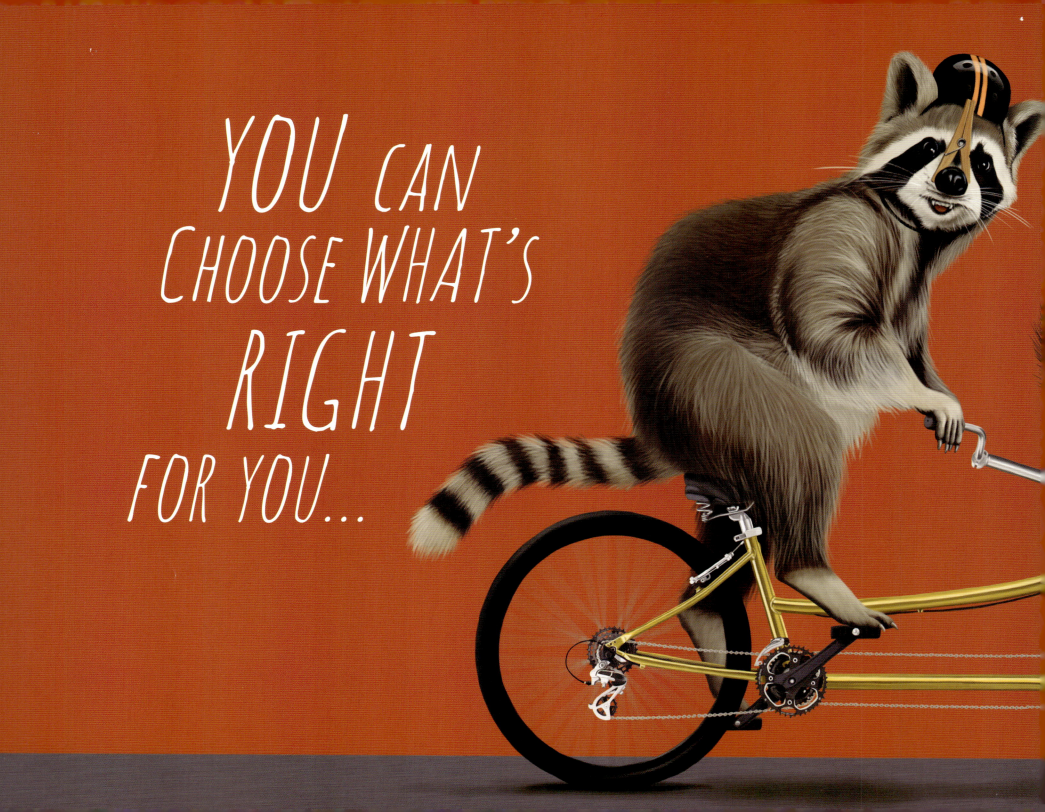

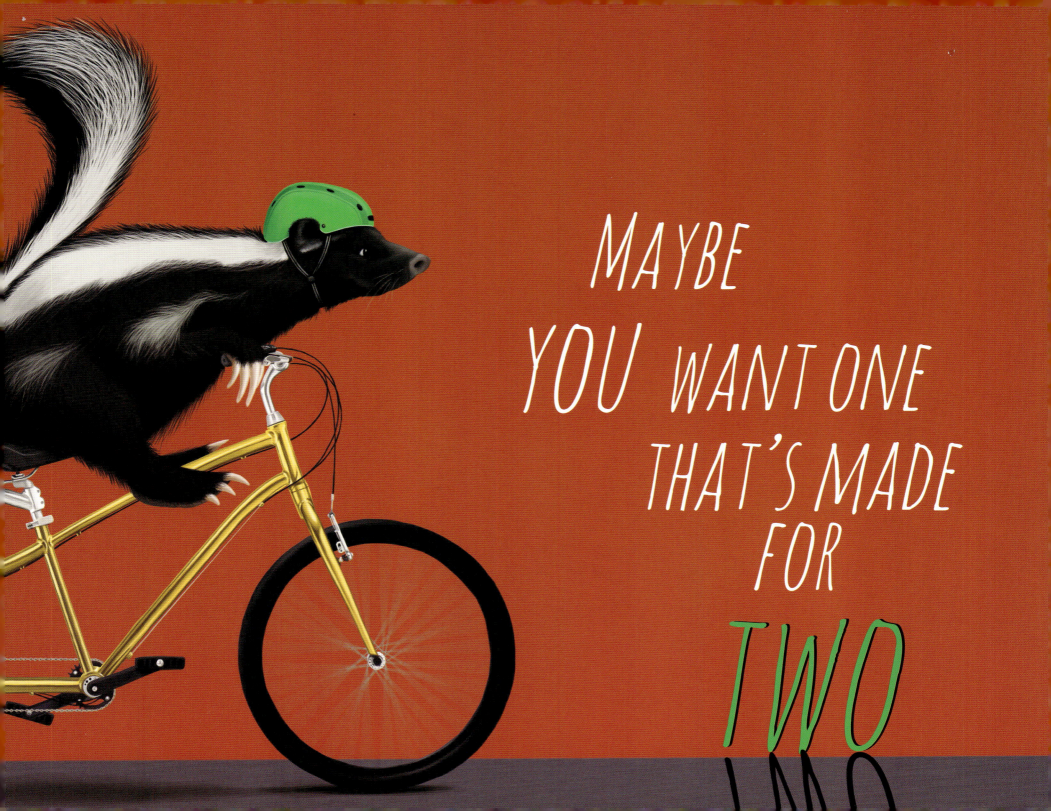

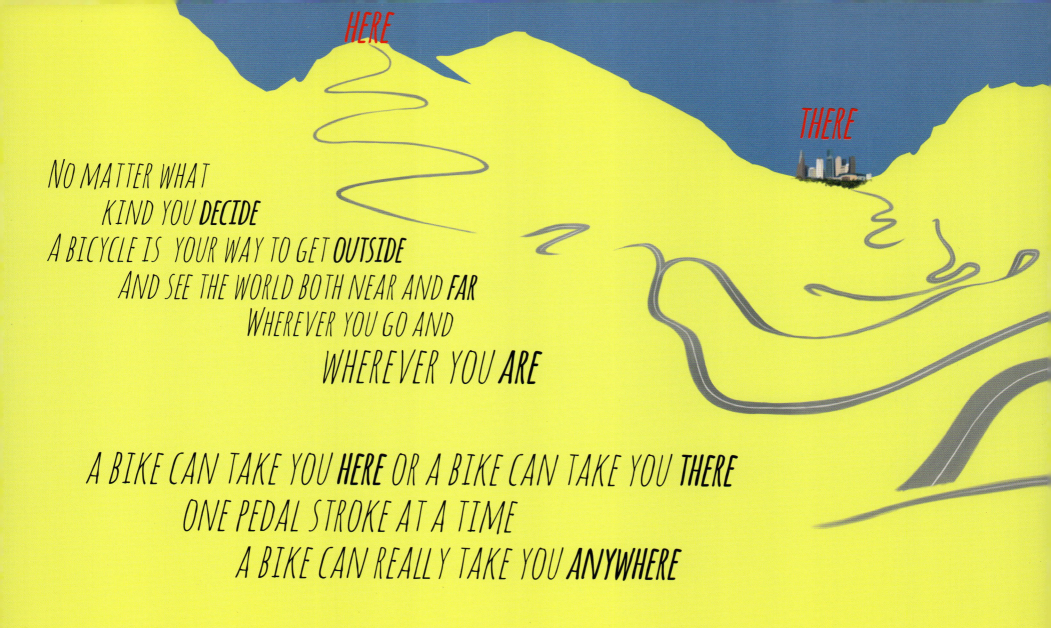

HERE

THERE

No matter what
kind you DECIDE
A bicycle is your way to get OUTSIDE
And see the world both near and FAR
Wherever you go and
WHEREVER YOU ARE

A BIKE CAN TAKE YOU HERE OR A BIKE CAN TAKE YOU THERE
ONE PEDAL STROKE AT A TIME
A BIKE CAN REALLY TAKE YOU ANYWHERE

BRING SOMETHING TO DRINK
AND HIT THE STREET

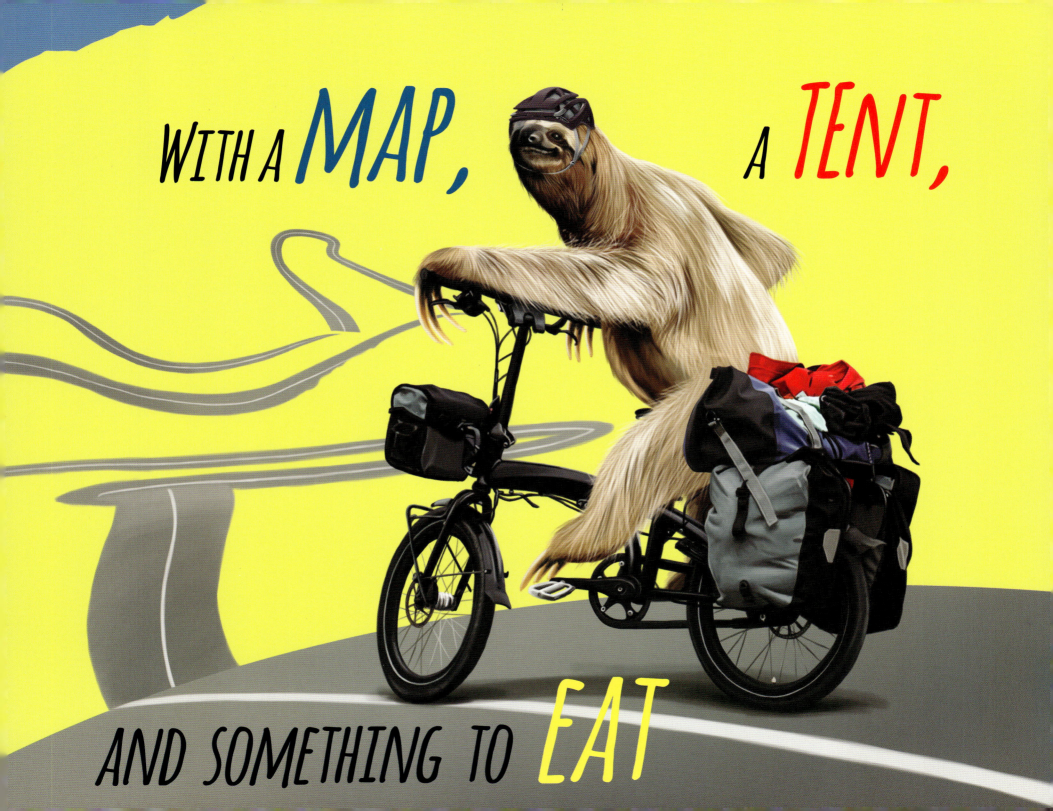

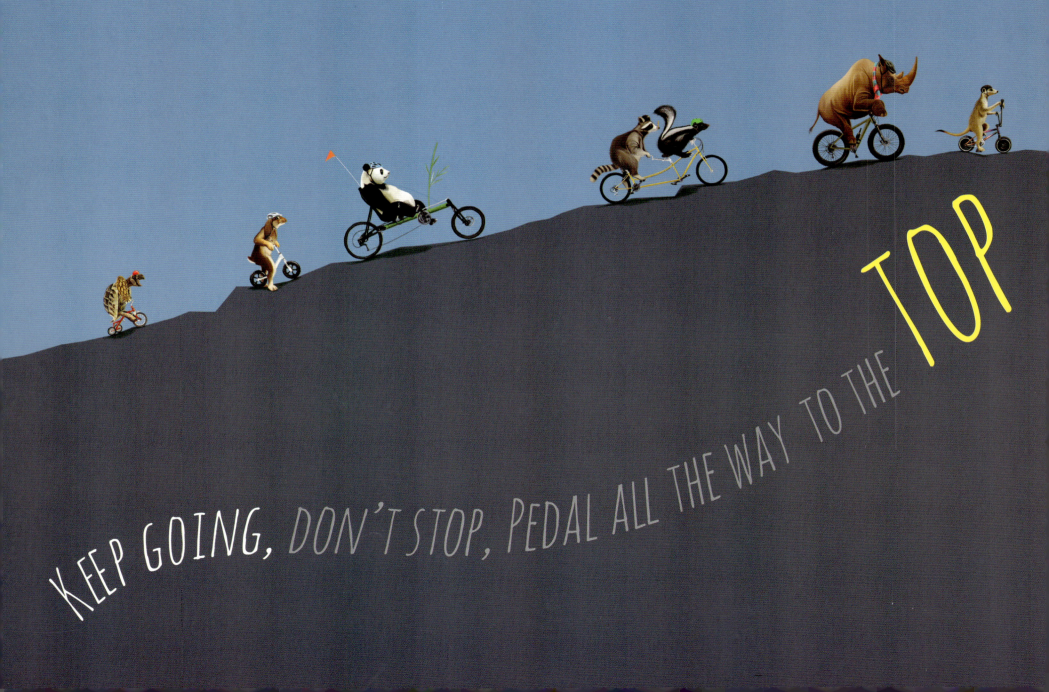

KEEP GOING, DON'T STOP, PEDAL ALL THE WAY TO THE TOP

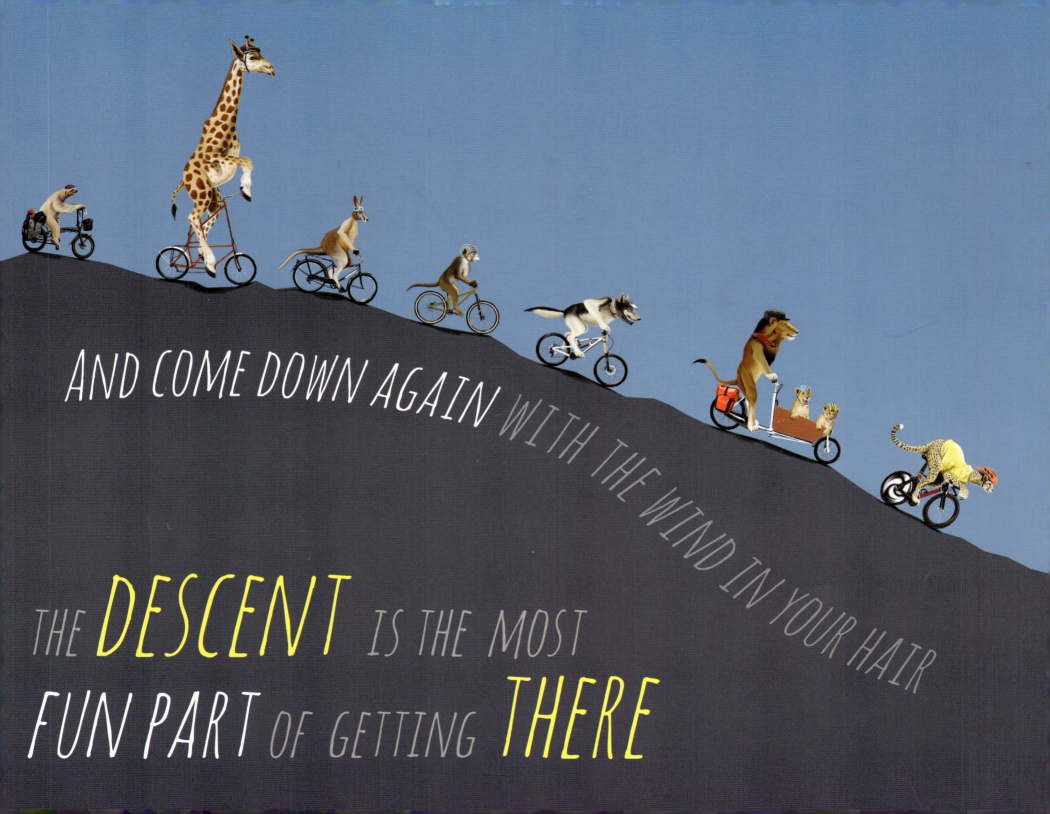

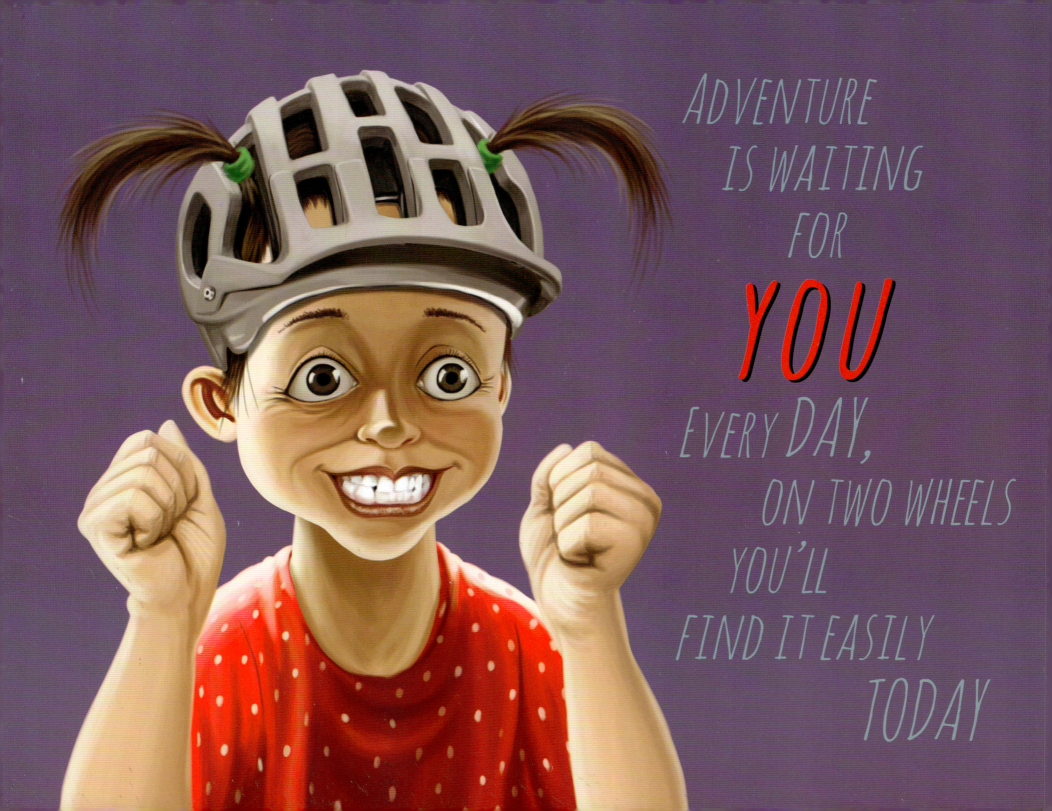

ADVENTURE
IS WAITING
FOR
YOU
EVERY DAY,
ON TWO WHEELS
YOU'LL
FIND IT EASILY
TODAY

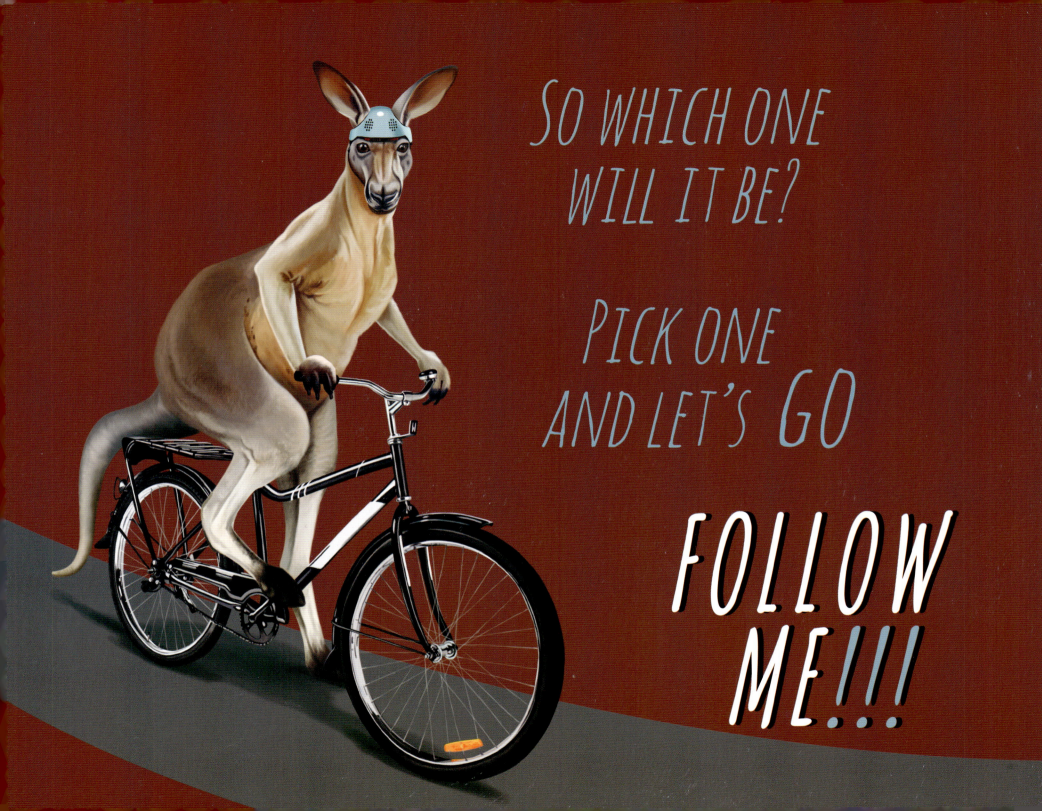

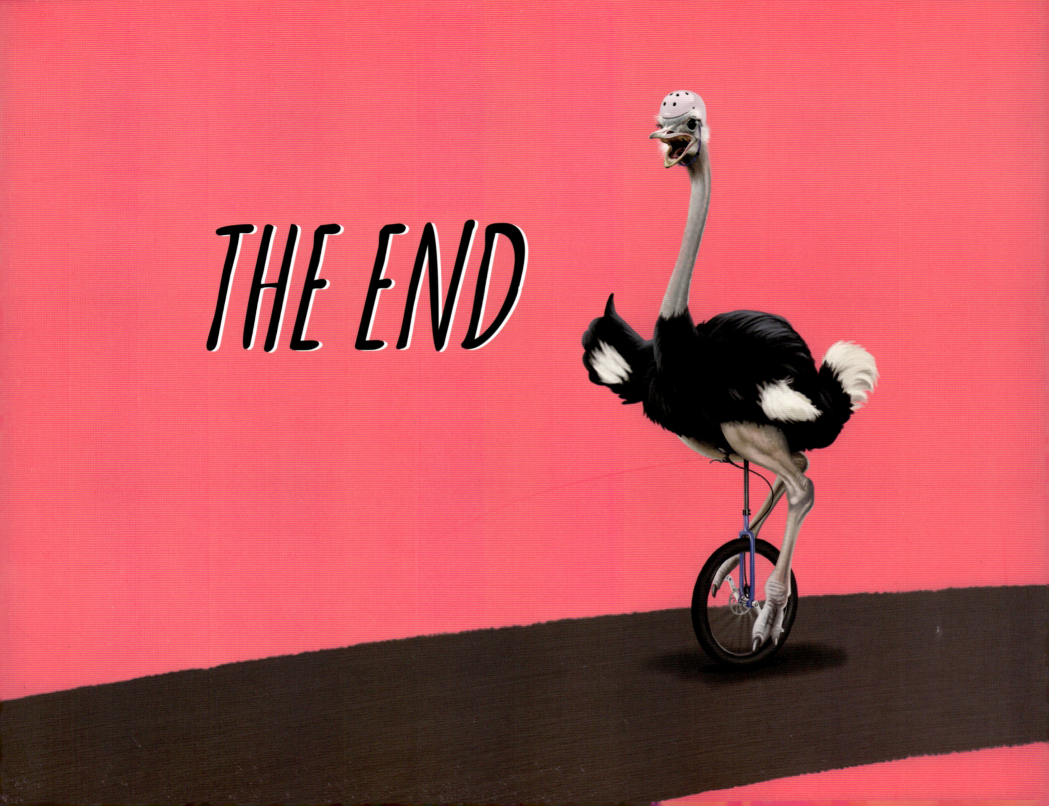

THIS BOOK WAS ART DIRECTED BY **HEIDI VOLPE** WHO'S LOVING TOUCH MADE EACH AND EVERY ONE OF THESE PAGES COME TO

LIFE!!!

THANK YOU TO ALL OF MY ORIGINAL **KICKSTARTER** BACKERS. WITHOUT YOUR GENEROUS SUPPORT, "A BIKE FOR YOU" WOULD NOT HAVE BECOME A REALITY!